The Easy Ways to Lose Weight

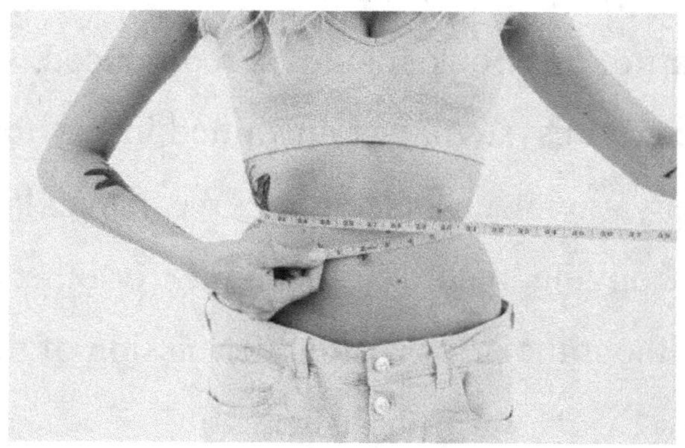

Transform Your Life with an Easy and Accessible Weight Loss Solution

Karen Waldrop

Table of Content

Hannah's Weight Loss Journey

For years, Hannah had struggled with her Weight. Despite trying every diet and fitness regimen, nothing appeared to work for her. She felt discouraged and disheartened, as if she could never accomplish her objectives.

She came across an article on The Easy Way to Lose Weight one day as she went through her social media. A regimen promising long-lasting benefits without drastic dieting or strenuous exercise appeared too good to be true. But she decided to try it because she needed a solution.

Compared to other programs she had tried, this one was quite different. She was instructed to adjust her lifestyle in subtle, enduring ways that would result in long-term weight reduction. They offered her instructions on preparing nutritious meals, making smart food choices, and simple workouts she could do at home.

Hannah was shocked by how soon she began to notice the effects. Without experiencing deprivation or fatigue, she was able to reduce Weight. She was even allowed to enjoy her favorite foods in moderation, which gave her the impression that she was still in charge of her course of action.

The Easy Way to Lose Weight gave Hannah the knowledge and inspiration to accomplish her objectives. She made long-lasting adjustments that allowed her to sustain her weight reduction and feel better than ever, both physically and psychologically. She felt really happy that the program had finally enabled her to discover the road to success.

Chapter 1: introduction

The problem with traditional weight loss methods

Losing weight may be a challenging and unpleasant journey for many individuals. Traditional weight reduction techniques can include stringent diets and strenuous exercise routines, which may be difficult to maintain over the long run. While these techniques may lead to initial weight loss, they frequently fail to deliver long-lasting results.

One of the primary issues with conventional weight reduction techniques is that they only emphasize calorie restriction and calorie expenditure via exercise. This method may work in the short term, but it only deals with the underlying factors leading to weight gains, such as bad eating habits and sedentary lifestyles.

Traditional weight loss techniques frequently advocate a "one size fits all" strategy, which might not be appropriate for everyone. Because every person has a unique body, what works for one person might not work for another. When conventional techniques don't provide the intended outcomes, this might result in emotions of dissatisfaction and failure.

Conventional weight reduction techniques may be time- and money-consuming is another issue. Exercise routines sometimes call for pricey gym memberships or specialty meals or supplements, and many diets do as well. Many individuals may find this a barrier to entrance, especially those with few resources or demanding schedules.

Last but not least, conventional weight reduction techniques may be emotionally stressful. When objectives are not achieved, restricting one's diet and pushing oneself to work out may be difficult and cause emotions of guilt and shame.

Why it isn't easy to lose weight

For many individuals, losing weight may be a difficult and unpleasant task. Even though losing weight is just a matter of eating less and exercising more, many things can make it challenging.

Our bodies are built to retain fat, which is one of the primary reasons why losing weight may be challenging. More fat reserves would boost the probability of survival during famine or food shortage. Therefore, this is an evolutionary response to such conditions. It implies that in reaction to a calorie shortage, our bodies may slow our metabolism or make us feel more hungry.

The contemporary lifestyle might also make losing weight challenging. Many of us lead sedentary lifestyles, spending countless hours in front of screens or at desks. Due to poor posture and muscular imbalances, it may be challenging to move and exercise properly and difficult to burn enough calories.

Processed foods, sugar, and unhealthy fats are frequently found in our modern diets, promoting weight gain and making it more difficult to lose weight. These foods often have a lot of calories but few nutrients, which causes overeating and inadequate satiety.

Several psychological and emotional factors can also make weight loss challenging. Stress, worry, and sadness may affect our eating behaviors, making it more difficult to maintain a good diet and exercise schedule. Fatigue and lack of sleep may make it more difficult to remain motivated and make good decisions.

The Approach of This Book

The approach of "The Easy Way to Lose Weight" is to tackle weight reduction holistically and sustainably, emphasizing lifestyle changes above temporary remedies. This book acknowledges that conventional weight reduction techniques might be difficult to follow and not provide long-term success.

The significance of making gradual, reasonable adjustments to one's lifestyle is instead emphasized throughout the book. This strategy acknowledges that losing weight requires patience, consistency, and dedication to produce long-lasting outcomes.

The book covers various issues, including how to grasp the fundamentals of weight reduction and the functions of calories and metabolism and create reasonable objectives and adopt long-lasting lifestyle changes. It also discusses the value of a balanced diet and frequent exercise and offers helpful advice on making better decisions and maintaining motivation.

The book also offers advice on measuring progress and finding community, promotes the value of responsibility and support, and underlines the necessity of assistance. The book also offers tactics for overcoming plateaus and keeping on track as typical obstacles and setbacks may arise throughout weight reduction.

The goal of "The Easy Way to Lose Weight" is to provide a doable, long-lasting, and tailored weight reduction method that considers distinct requirements and preferences. With the aid of this book, readers will be able to lose weight and enhance their general health and well-being in a fun and long-lasting manner.

Chapter 2: Understanding Weight Loss

The basics of weight loss

You must establish a calorie deficit, or burn more calories than you consume, to lose weight. Your body begins to burn fat reserves for energy when a calorie deficit results in weight loss.

A few fundamental ideas form the basis of effective weight loss:

- **Calories in, calories out: As** previously noted, achieving a calorie deficit is the key to losing weight. According to this, it would help to expend more calories than you consume. You may either eat less or walk more to achieve this.

- Your body consumes calories at a certain pace at rest, known as metabolism. It includes the calories your body expends to keep breathing and pumping blood. Some individuals burn more calories at rest than others due to their higher metabolisms. However, you can increase your metabolism by training in strength to gain muscle.

- **Food caloric content:** Calories are not all created equal. It's important to consider the food's quality as well. You may feel satiated for longer if you eat foods rich in fiber, protein, and healthy fats. On the other hand, foods that are heavy in sugar and harmful fats tend to be full and might result in overeating.

- **Exercise:** While it is possible to lose weight via dietary changes, physical activity may help you burn more calories and enhance your general health. In contrast to strength training, which may help you gain muscle and speed up your metabolism, cardiovascular activity (such as running, cycling, or swimming) can burn many calories.

Consistency is the most crucial element in effective weight reduction. Instead of depending on short-term diets or fast remedies, sustainable weight reduction involves implementing long-term lifestyle adjustments. Finding a sustainable and pleasurable method of eating and exercising is necessary, and it must be followed over time.

How calories work

Calories are units of energy used to calculate how much energy is in food and how much energy your body expends each day. When you eat, your body digests the food's proteins, fats, and carbohydrates to produce energy in the form of calories. Then, your body uses this energy to carry out all its processes, such as breathing, blood circulation, and muscle movement.

Various variables, including age, gender, height, weight, and amount of exercise, influence your daily calorie requirements. The quantity of calories your body burns when at rest is known as your basal metabolic rate (BMR). The bulk of the calories you burn daily come from your BMR, but you also burn calories during exercise and the digestion and absorption of meals.

Your body will store extra calories as fat if you take in more than it uses up, which might eventually result in weight gain. However, if you burn more calories than you take in, your body will start to use the fat stored as fuel, resulting in weight loss.

Remember that not all calories are created equally. The caloric intake and expenditure are crucial for weight control, but so is the caliber of the food you consume. It may be simpler to adhere to a healthy diet if you eat foods rich in fiber, protein, and healthy fats since they tend to be more satiating and may prolong your sensation of fullness. On the other hand, foods that are heavy in sugar and harmful fats tend to be full and might result in overeating.

The part metabolism plays

The metabolism is important for controlling weight and maintaining general health. The term "metabolism" describes the chemical reactions in your body to support life, including transforming food into energy. The pace at which your body uses calories to carry out these functions is known as your metabolic rate.

Your age, gender, genetics, body composition, and lifestyle choices are just a few of the variables that might influence your metabolic rate. For instance, those with greater muscle tend to have higher metabolic rates because muscular tissue consumes more calories at rest than fat tissue.

Calorie balance is a critical idea that affects weight control about metabolism. Your body will store extra calories as fat if you take in more than it uses up, which might eventually result in weight gain. However, if you burn more calories than you take in, your body will start to use the fat stored as fuel, resulting in weight loss.

Certain meals and lifestyle choices may impact your metabolism. Because protein takes more energy to digest than carbohydrates or fat, eating a high-protein diet, for instance, can increase metabolism. On the other hand, crash dieting or substantially limiting your calorie intake might cause your metabolism to slow down since your body will attempt to preserve energy because it will believe that you are starving.

The metabolism contributes to general health in addition to helping people control their weight. For instance, it has been shown that a slow metabolism increases the risk of type 2 diabetes, but a quick metabolism reduces the risk of heart disease.

The importance of exercise

Exercise, including a healthy weight, is crucial for maintaining overall health and well-being. Numerous health advantages of regular exercise include:

- **Calorie burning:** Burning calories via exercise is crucial for maintaining a healthy weight. You establish a calorie deficit by burning more calories than you take in, which results in weight reduction.

- Strength training, in particular, may help you gain and maintain muscle mass. More muscle may raise your metabolic rate and help you burn more calories throughout the day since muscle tissue burns more calories at rest than fat tissue.

- **Increasing metabolism:** Exercise may increase your metabolism after you stop working out. Resistance and high-intensity interval training (HIIT) have been demonstrated to have the strongest effects on increasing metabolism.

- **Increasing insulin sensitivity:** Exercising may help you have better insulin sensitivity, crucial for controlling your blood sugar and lowering your risk of type 2 diabetes.

- **Reducing inflammation:** Inflammation in the body, connected to several chronic illnesses, may be reduced by exercise.

- **Enhancing mood:** Studies have shown that exercise may improve mood and lessen depressive and anxious symptoms.

- Enhancing cardiovascular health: By fortifying the heart and enhancing blood flow, exercise helps to promote cardiovascular health.

Exercise may be a terrific method to reduce stress, enhance sleep, and improve the overall quality of life in addition to these physical advantages. It is advised to strive for at least 150 minutes of moderate-intensity aerobic activity or 75 minutes of vigorous-intensity aerobic activity each week and strength training activities at least twice per week to enjoy the advantages of exercise.

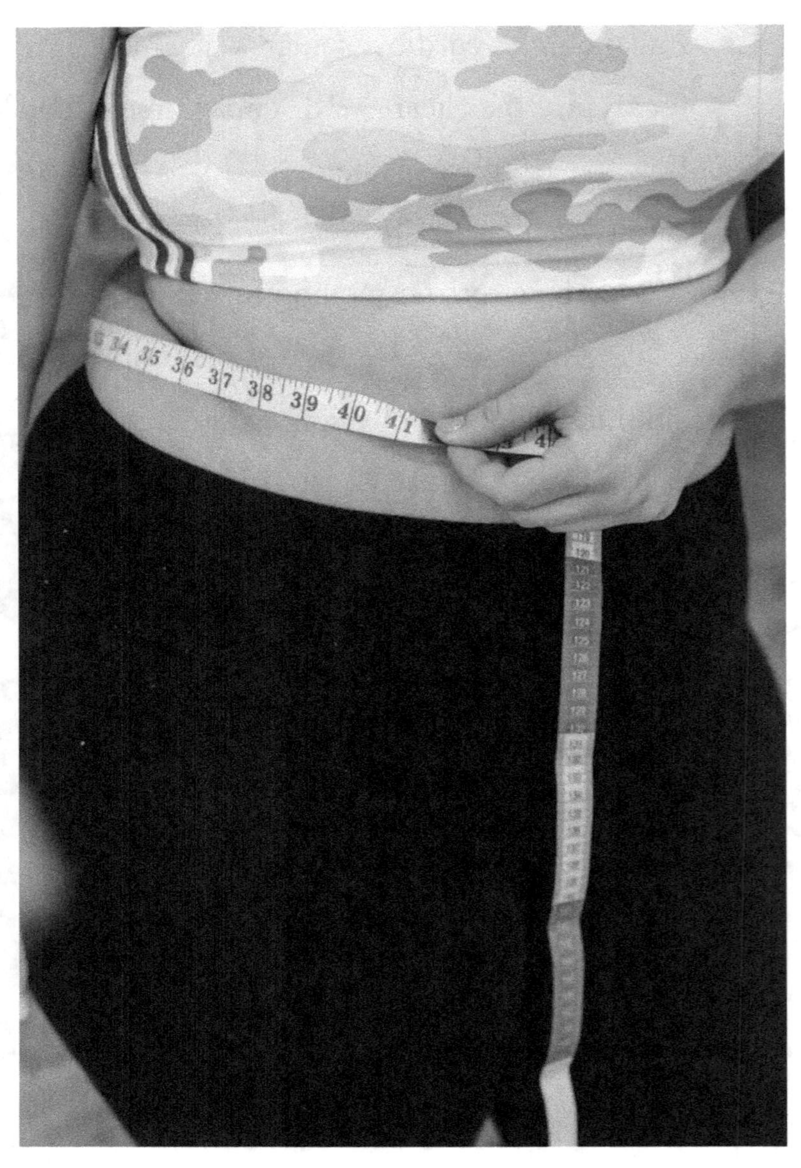

21 | THE EASY WAYS TO LOSE WEIGHT

Chapter 3: Setting Realistic Goals

Why setting realistic goals is important

setting attainable objectives is essential for successful weight reduction. While setting high standards and aiming for quick weight loss may be alluring, these strategies can be unsustainable and even harmful in the long run. Setting realistic objectives is crucial for weight reduction for the following reasons:

Progress sustained over time will likely be made when realistic objectives are stated. The likelihood of maintaining weight reduction via healthy lifestyle modifications is higher than drastic efforts to achieve quick weight loss.

- **Avoid disappointment:** if you establish unattainable objectives and fail to meet them, you risk becoming depressed and giving up on your attempt to lose weight. You'll be more likely to observe improvement and steer clear of disappointment if you create attainable objectives.

- **Accomplishing modest goals can be rewarding:** Doable objectives help boost drive and self-assurance. It might encourage you to continue making good decisions and being dedicated to your weight reduction program.

- **Tension reduction:** setting improbable objectives might lead to unneeded tension and anxiety. You may lessen stress and take pleasure in weight reduction by establishing realistic objectives.

- **Focusing on health:** when you adjust your lifestyle to improve your overall health, rather than just striving to reach a specific weight target, you may concentrate on improving your health by setting realistic objectives.

It's crucial to consider your present habits and lifestyle and any health issues or physical restrictions you may have while establishing weight reduction objectives. You may get assistance from a registered dietitian or other healthcare professional in developing attainable objectives and a specific action plan. You may accomplish lasting weight reduction and enhance your general health and well-being by establishing attainable objectives and concentrating on healthy behaviors.

How to Set Achievable Goals

Setting realistic objectives is crucial for successful weight reduction. Setting realistic objectives can increase your chances of making long-term, sustainable improvements, boosting confidence, and preventing disappointment. Here are some pointers for establishing reasonable objectives for weight loss:

Set a clear and specific goal at the outset. Instead of choosing a broad goal, such as "lose weight," be more specific about what you want to accomplish. You may write, "Lose 10 pounds in 12 weeks" or "Reduce my body fat percentage by 5%." this aids in progress monitoring and motivational support.

Establish a reasonable timeline: While a goal is important, it's also crucial to establish a reasonable timeline for achieving it. Although it may be alluring, rapid weight loss can be unsustainable and harmful. Aim to lose 1-2 pounds of weight gradually each week.

Set smaller, more manageable goals: instead of concentrating only on the result, set smaller, more manageable goals. Consider dropping 2-3 pounds weekly if your objective is to shed 20 pounds. It might give you motivation and momentum.

Think about your habits and way of life while making goals: it's important to consider your routine. For instance, aiming for an hour of exercise may be unreasonable if you have a hectic schedule. Instead, make it a point to exercise for 30 minutes on most days of the week.

Be adaptable, while having a plan is vital, it's also crucial to be adaptable and ready to change your objectives. Due to the unpredictability of life, there may be moments when your efforts to lose weight stop or you encounter unforeseen difficulties. Be prepared to modify your objectives and strategy to remain on course.

Celebrate your accomplishments along the road, no matter how tiny, to show that you are making progress. The process of losing weight may become more fun. As a result, boosting confidence and drive.

Last, consider getting assistance from a licensed dietician or other medical professional or enrolling in a group that helps people lose weight. A support network helps keep you responsible, motivated, and on track to reach your objectives.

You may accomplish lasting weight reduction and enhance your general health and well-being by establishing attainable objectives and concentrating on healthy behaviors. Remember to be patient, adaptable, and recognize your accomplishments as you go.

The Benefits of Small Victories

Small accomplishments can have a big impact when it comes to losing weight. Gaining momentum toward achieving bigger objectives may be facilitated by hitting smaller milestones. Here are some advantages of acknowledging modest achievements in weight loss:

- **Increasing motivation:** Achieving a minor achievement, like slipping into clothes you previously couldn't fit into or finishing a workout without becoming out of breath, may give you a sense of satisfaction and increase your drive. It might encourage you to continue making good decisions and being dedicated to your weight reduction program.

- **Confidence-building:** Small triumphs may boost your belief in making wise decisions and realizing your objectives. It can assist you in overcoming obstacles and keeping your attention on the greater goal.

- Celebrating modest successes promotes constructive routines and attitudes. You're more likely to keep up a habit if, for instance, you reward yourself for drinking more water each day.

- Celebrating little triumphs might aid in tracking your progress toward greater objectives. You can notice your progress and maintain your motivation by concentrating on minor victories along the road.

- **Lowering stress:** Losing weight may sometimes be daunting and unpleasant. Small wins should be celebrated because they can ease stress and give a sense of relief and accomplishment.

- **Making the trip more enjoyable:** Highlighting little successes may add enjoyment and satisfaction to losing weight. You may cultivate a more positive outlook and take pleasure in achieving your objectives by concentrating on your successes.

Beyond weight reduction, good habits and behaviors promoting general health and well-being can also be reinforced by celebrating modest triumphs.

Small victories in weight loss can be as simple as drinking more water, experimenting with a new healthy recipe, getting more active daily, and reducing portion sizes. Create a pleasant and inspiring atmosphere for achieving greater weight reduction objectives by acknowledging and applauding these little accomplishments.

Small victories can have a significant impact on the success of weight loss. You may increase motivation, increase self-confidence, establish healthy habits, monitor progress, lower stress, enjoy the trip, and enhance your overall health and well-being by acknowledging tiny victories along the road.

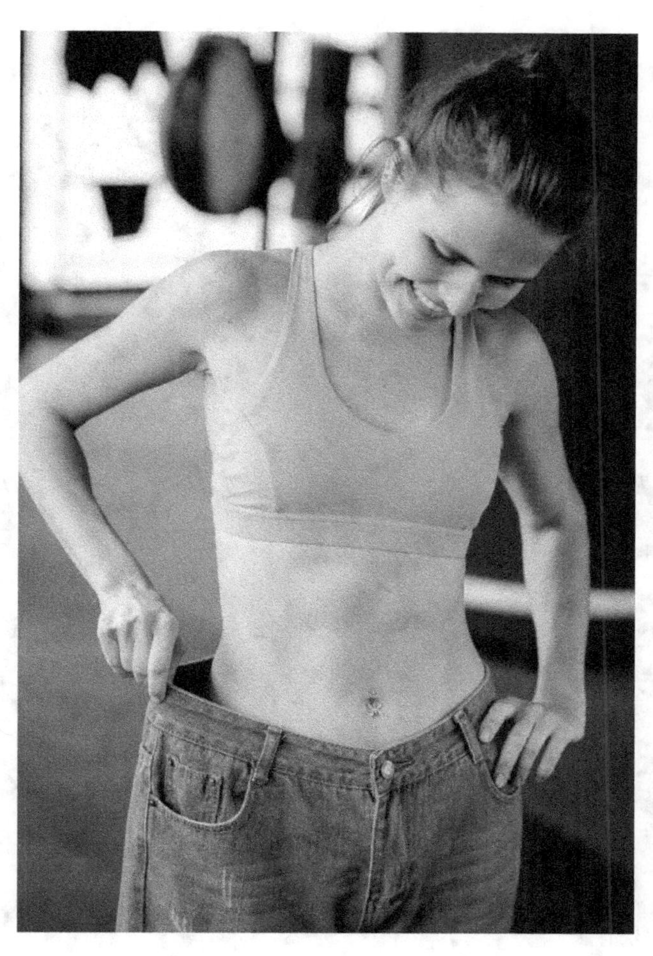

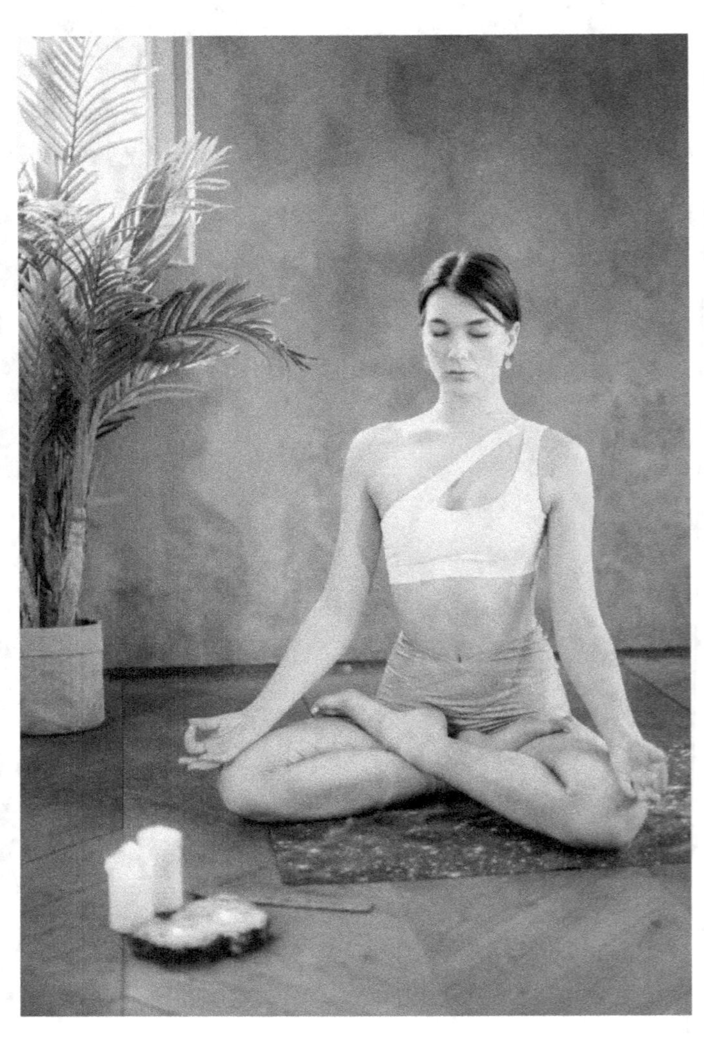

Chapter 4: Making Lifestyle Changes

How to Make Sustainable Lifestyle Changes

Making permanent lifestyle adjustments is key to long-term weight reduction and enhancing general health and well-being. Here are some pointers for changing to a sustainable lifestyle:

Try to make only a few adjustments at a time; this may be daunting and unsustainable. Instead, start small. Start by implementing simple, easy-to-maintain adjustments, like increasing the number of fruits and vegetables in your diet or going for regular walks.

Set attainable goals:

Be honest while determining what you can accomplish.

Avoid setting yourself up for failure by attempting too much too soon.

Establish attainable objectives that you can maintain over time.

- **Change slowly:** gradual adjustments are simpler to maintain than abrupt, severe ones. For instance, decreasing portion sizes in half at once may not be as sustainable as gradually over time.

- **Don't just think about losing weight:** think about actions that will help you lose weight, such as increasing your vegetable intake, water intake, or physical exercise.

- **Identify any roadblocks:** such as a hectic schedule or a lack of support, that may keep you from adopting lasting lifestyle changes. Seek assistance to help you overcome these challenges or find ways to get around them.

- **Celebrate minor triumphs:** like achieving a daily step target or attempting a new healthy meal, as they come along the road. Small victories should be celebrated to increase motivation and reinforce good behavior.

- **Keep yourself accountable:** by documenting your food consumption, exercising regularly, or seeking the aid of a buddy or accountability partner.

- **Establish a support network:** A support network may assist you in remaining motivated and responsible. Consider joining a support group for those trying to lose weight, or ask a personal trainer or licensed dietician for assistance.

You may lose weight permanently and enhance your general health and well-being by making tiny, steady adjustments and concentrating on sustainable habits. Remember to be patient and nice to yourself and appreciate your tiny accomplishments as you go along.

Tips for Incorporating Healthier Habits

Although incorporating healthier habits into your daily routine can be difficult, losing weight permanently and improving your general health and well-being is necessary. Here are some pointers for developing better lifestyle habits:

Plan: Establish clear objectives and develop a strategy for achieving them. Make a strategy outlining the measures you'll take to attain your objectives and write them down.

Only attempt to implement a few changes at a time; start modestly. Start small by increasing your water intake or adding a regular stroll to your schedule, and work your way up.

Make it fun: Finding methods to make healthy behaviors entertaining might make them more pleasurable. For instance, try a new, nutritious cuisine or locate a workout partner to make exercise more fun.

Think positively: Concentrate on the good adjustments you're making and the advantages they'll bring rather than what you can't have or must give up.

Be dependable: When it comes to implementing better behaviors, consistency is crucial. Make sure to incorporate these routines into your day and maintain them despite difficulties.

To keep accountable and motivated, seek assistance from friends, family, or a support group.

You may also see a personal trainer or licensed dietician for added assistance and direction.

Track your development: Keeping tabs on your development will help you remain inspired and recognize your progress. Keep a food diary, log your workouts, or use a fitness app to measure your progress.

Celebrate your accomplishments: Take time to recognize each step-by-step victory, such as losing a certain amount of weight or finishing an exercise. Celebrating these victories may encourage beneficial behaviors and increase motivation.

Incorporating healthy behaviors into your daily routine may take some time and work, but the rewards are worthwhile. You may make long-lasting changes that will assist you in reaching your weight reduction goals and enhancing your general health and well-being by beginning small, creating a plan, getting support, and celebrating victories.

Consistency Is Important

Consistency is crucial when it comes to losing weight and forming healthy habits since it enables you to gain momentum and advance over time. Consistency is crucial for the following reasons.

Establishing healthy habits regularly over time might aid in forming new habits. Maintaining habits over the long run is simpler since they are automatic actions that don't require much thinking or effort.

Builds momentum, Being consistent aids in creating momentum, which makes it simpler to carry on moving toward your objectives. Maintaining good habits when you do it regularly gets simpler, which may promote future growth and success.

A feeling of success is generated when you continuously practice healthy actions, which also perpetuates good habits. It may make it simpler to keep moving forward by boosting drive and confidence.

Prevents setbacks by building a solid foundation of good behaviors. Consistency may assist in avoiding setbacks. Consistency in your healthy activities makes fending off temptations and getting beyond potential challenges simpler.

Progress may be made gradually thanks to consistency, which is more enduring than abrupt, extreme changes. Your weight reduction objectives may advance by making gradual, incremental modifications.

Controls your actions and makes you feel more in control of your weight loss journey: Consistency gives you control over your behaviors. You're more likely to feel in control of your development and empowered when you're consistent with your healthy behaviors.

Consistency is key when it comes to losing weight and forming healthy habits. You may form habits, generate momentum, feel more in control of your weight loss journey, avoid setbacks, and achieve steady progress by persistently participating in healthy activities over time.

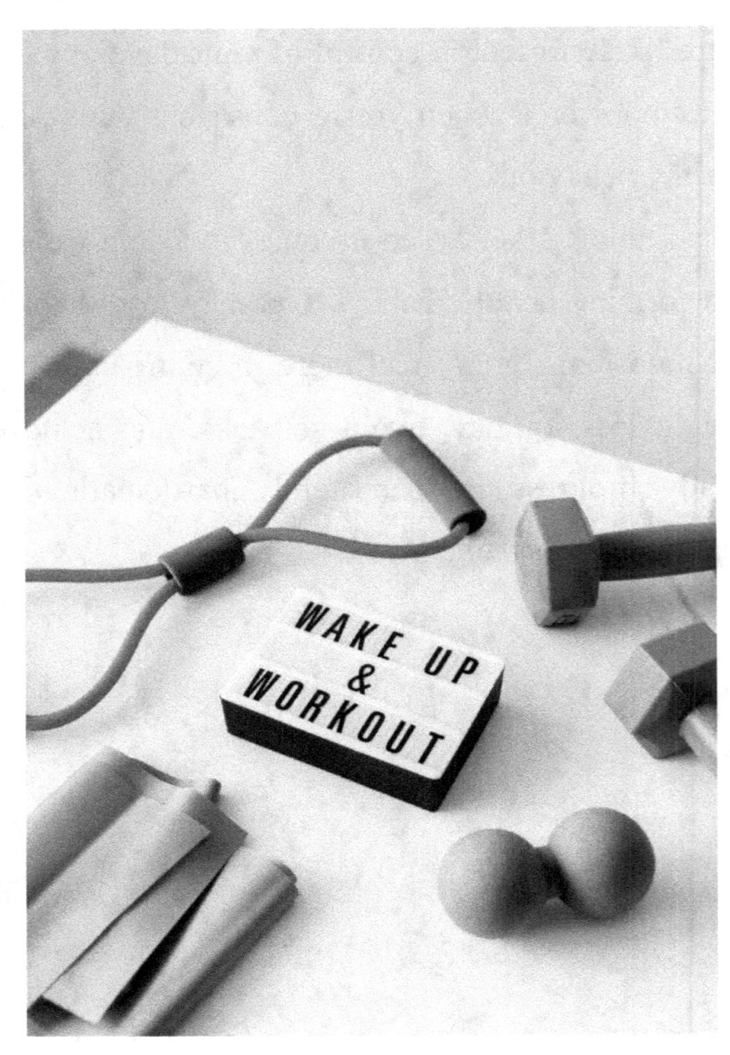

WAKE UP
&
WORKOUT

Chapter 5: Eating for Weight Loss

Understanding Portion Control

A key component of diet maintenance and weight reduction is portion management. It describes eating a certain quantity of food to satisfy your body's nutritional requirements without overindulging or ingesting excessive calories. The following are some crucial concepts about portion control:

- **Serving size and portion size:** Serving size refers to the quantity of food advised to be consumed and shown on the nutrition label. Portion size refers to the amount of food that you eat. To prevent overeating, one should practice moderation. , it's important to be aware of the ideal serving size and to measure or estimate your quantities.

- **Use measurement tools:** To ensure you're eating the proper serving size, use measuring cups, a food scale, or other equipment to measure your amounts precisely. It is crucial for items like nuts, chips, and sweets that are simple to overeat.

- **Observe your body:** Pay attention to your hunger and fullness indicators to decide how much food you need. When you're satiated but not overstuffed, stop eating. You may learn to listen to your body's cues by eating slowly and carefully.

- Pick foods high in vitamins, minerals, and fiber that are nutrient-dense. When portioning your meals, keep this in mind. These meals provide your body with the nutrition it needs to operate correctly while also helping you feel satiated for longer.

- **Eat out with awareness:** Restaurant portions are frequently larger than recommended serving sizes, so paying attention to how much food you're consuming is crucial. To help you manage your quantities, think about sharing a meal or bringing leftovers home.

- **Utilize visual cues:** Visual cues can help you choose the right portion sizes. For instance, a portion of vegetables should be the size of your fist, and a serving of protein should be comparable to a deck of cards.

- **In advance:** You can control your portion sizes and choose healthful foods by organizing your meals. You're less prone to overeat or make rash judgments if you have a strategy.

- **Make sure to eat meals:** Eating frequently throughout the day is vital since skipping meals might result in overeating later in the day. By doing so, you may avoid overeating and maintain a healthy metabolism.

- **Eat mindfully:** Mindful eating is being present and conscious of your food choices, appreciating your meal, and paying attention to your hunger and fullness indicators. It will encourage more conscious eating, which can improve portion management.

- **Use smaller dishes and plates:** You may more easily manage your servings using smaller bowls and plates. Your mind may think you need less food when your plate seems full. Slowing your meals will help you understand when you're full using smaller utensils.

The Role of Macronutrients

Carbohydrates, proteins, and lipids are the three nutrients the body needs in substantial quantities to operate correctly. Each macronutrient has a special function in the body and is necessary to maintain general health and reach weight reduction objectives.

However, not all carbohydrates are created equal. They are necessary for physical exertion and fuel the muscles, brain, and other organs. Not all forms of carbohydrates are the same. Simple carbs, such as those in soda and sweets, may cause blood sugar to rise and fall rapidly. The more fiber-rich and sustained-energy complex carbs, such as those in whole grains, fruits, and vegetables, are a superior option.

The body depends on proteins to build and repair tissues. They are crucial for preserving lean muscle mass and bolstering the immune system. A few examples of foods high in protein include meat, chicken, fish, eggs, beans, and nuts.

Fats: Fats are necessary for the body to absorb vitamins and minerals and insulate and cushion the organs. But not all fats are made equally. Because they can raise cholesterol levels and increase the risk of heart disease, saturated and trans fats should be consumed in moderation. Unsaturated fats, including those in nuts, seeds, and fatty fish, are preferable because they are healthier.

It's crucial to consider your diet's macronutrient composition to reach your weight reduction objectives. Despite the significance of each macronutrient, it is crucial to maintain a balance between them. A macronutrient may be consumed excessively to cause weight gain and other health issues. You may promote overall health and reach your weight reduction goals with a balanced diet that includes a range of complete foods, such as fruits, vegetables, whole grains, lean proteins, and healthy fats.

Making Healthier Food Choices

Achieving and maintaining a healthy weight requires making better dietary choices. Here are some pointers to assist you in choosing healthier foods:

Emphasize whole, nutrient-rich foods: Whole foods have undergone little processing and are rich in different types of nutrients. Fruits, vegetables, whole grains, lean meats, and healthy fats are a few of them. As the cornerstone of your diet, choose these items.

Please pay attention to portion sizes since they may significantly affect your calorie consumption. Until you can accurately estimate portion sizes, measure your food with measuring cups, spoons, or a scale.

Limit added sugars and refined carbs since they may cause blood sugar to surge and lead to weight gain. These substances are often found in processed meals and sugary beverages. Limit processed foods with added sugars and refined carbs and opt for whole foods.

Pick lean proteins: Lean proteins have fewer calories and fat than their higher-fat counterparts. Examples of lean proteins include chicken, turkey, fish, and legumes. They are crucial for gaining and maintaining muscle mass.

Be careful how much fat you consume. Limit saturated and trans fats and choose good fats like those in nuts, seeds, and fatty fish.

Stay hydrated by drinking plenty of water, which can make you feel full and help you avoid overeating. Aim for 8 cups of water or more each day.

Be conscious of your eating patterns since doing so may lead to better food choices.

Strategies for Dining Out

Eating out might be difficult when trying to lose weight, but it doesn't have to stop you from making progress. Here are some tips to assist you in choosing healthier options while eating out:

In advance: Check out the menu online before visiting the restaurant to see the options. Avoid foods fried or smothered in creamy sauces, and look for meals that are lower in calories and fat.

Consider splitting a dish or taking half of your dinner home since restaurant servings are sometimes far greater than you need. You may also order an appetizer as your main entrée or request a half-portion.

Customize your order: Be bold and request changes or alterations. Choose grilled or baked alternatives over fried ones, and request dressings, sauces, and garnishes on the side.

Start with a salad: By filling up on fiber-rich and low-calorie veggies at the beginning of your meal, you may consume less food overall.

Watch what you drink: Extra calories from drinks might creep up on you. Avoid sugary beverages, alcohol, and high-calorie coffee drinks in favor of water, unsweetened tea, or other low-calorie choices.

Be conscious of how you eat. Savor each mouthful and eat carefully. Consider your signs of hunger and fullness. Even if food is left on your plate, stop eating when full.

You may enjoy eating out without jeopardizing your efforts to lose weight by using the below-mentioned tactics. Remember that it's OK to splurge sometimes, but concentrate on making good decisions most of the time.

Chapter 6: Exercising for Weight Loss

The Benefits of Exercise for Weight Loss

Any weight loss program must include exercise because it offers several advantages that can aid in achieving and maintaining a healthy weight. The following are a few advantages of exercise for weight loss:

Exercise helps you burn calories: which might help you reduce your calorie intake and lose weight. Your body composition, weight, activity style, and intensity affect how many calories you burn.

Increases metabolism: Regular exercise helps speed up your body's calorie-burning process, or metabolism. Even when you aren't exercising, this may help you burn extra calories.

The lean muscle mass may be developed by resistance training, including bodyweight movements and weightlifting. Muscle burns more calories at rest than fat because it has a higher metabolic activity. Your body burns more calories throughout the day, and you have more lean muscle mass.

Enhances cardiovascular health: By fortifying your heart and lungs, cardiovascular activity like jogging, cycling, or swimming may enhance cardiovascular health. You can exercise longer and burn more calories as a result.

Exercise may help people feel less stressed and anxious, which helps prevent them from overeating and gaining weight. Regular exercise may also lift your spirits and give you more energy.

Exercise may help you sleep better, which benefits weight reduction and general health. Getting adequate sleep may assist in balancing hormones that impact metabolism and hunger.

Regular exercise might assist you in maintaining your weight reduction by avoiding weight gain. Additionally, it can assist you in forming wholesome routines and a favorable attitude toward physical activity and exercise.

You may take advantage of these advantages and reach your weight reduction objectives more successfully by including regular exercise in your weight loss regimen. To avoid injury and fatigue, always remember to begin carefully and gradually increase the intensity and length of your exercises.

How to Choose a Training Regimen You Like

You must choose a training regimen you love to maintain your fitness objectives and make exercise a regular part of your life. The following advice may help you discover an exercise regimen that you enjoy:

- **Try a variety of exercises:** Try out various workouts, such as yoga, weightlifting, jogging, or dancing courses. It's alright if you discover that you prefer certain hobbies to others.

- **Think about your preferences:** Consider your favorite pastimes, such as participating in a group, going outside, or listening to music. Look for workouts that cater to these inclinations, such as dancing classes with cheerful music or outdoor boot camps.

- **Find a fitness partner:** Exercising with a friend or family member can make it more fun and keep you accountable. It may also be an enjoyable social pastime.

- It might get monotonous to follow the same training program every day. Try new workouts or add variety to your routine to change things.

- Goal-setting may help you stay motivated by giving you something to strive towards, such as finishing a 5k or learning a new yoga posture.

- **Consider a personal trainer:** You may create a fitness plan specific to your objectives and preferences with a personal trainer. They may also provide direction and encouragement to keep you motivated.

- **Feel free to alter:** If an exercise is too unpleasant or challenging, alter it to make it more tolerable. If running isn't your thing, try walking or jogging instead.

- Remember that discovering a training regimen you love may take some time and experimentation. You'll ultimately discover a program that you enjoy, and that helps you reach your fitness objectives if you're patient and have an open mind.

Tips on Staying Motivated

It might not be easy to stay motivated while attempting to lose weight. Here are some ideas to help you stay motivated and on course:

- **Set attainable, defined objectives:** by being realistic about them. Setting impossible standards may cause irritation and demotivation.

- **Celebrate your accomplishments:** as you go along, even the little ones. Every pound dropped, every wholesome habit created, and each exercise finished is a step closer to your objective. Please spend some time appreciating and honoring their achievements.

- **Find a system of support:** Be in the company of individuals who support and encourage your aspirations. Find a workout partner, enroll in a support group for people trying to lose weight, or hire a personal trainer.

- **Establish a routine:** Create a schedule that works for you and follow it religiously. The secret to attaining your weight reduction objectives is consistency.

- **Reward yourself by creating a system of rewards for achieving your objectives:** Pick non-food incentives like a massage, a new workout outfit, or a night out with friends.

- **Utilize a weight loss journal or an app to keep track of your progress:** Observing your progress can help you stay inspired.

- Visualize yourself succeeding by imagining how it would feel to achieve your objective. This inspirational image might help you stay motivated and concentrated.

- **Change your routine:** by doing new exercises, including various nutritious foods in your diet, or discovering new methods to keep active. Variety can keep things fresh and avoid becoming monotonous.

Remember that maintaining motivation is a process, and setbacks are common. Never give up, remain committed to your objectives, and go on moving in the direction of a healthy way of life.

Chapter 7: Staying Accountable

The Importance of Tracking Progress

It might not be easy to lose weight, and it takes a lot of focus and attention. Your nutrition, exercise regimen, sleeping patterns, and stress levels are just a few of the variables that might impact your weight reduction efforts. Tracking your progress is an essential component that impacts your ability to reach your weight reduction objectives. In this article, we'll look at why keeping track of your progress is crucial for weight reduction.

You may see patterns and trends in your development that can impede your attempts to lose weight. You can see areas where you may need to improve or where you need to make changes if you keep track of what you eat, how much you exercise, and other pertinent information. You could see, for instance, that you consume more calories on the weekends or that your sleeping habits influence your hunger. You may modify your schedule and remain on track by being aware of this.

Monitoring your development may keep you responsible and motivated. Seeing your progress and how far you've come may be inspiring and motivating. On the other side, if you are having trouble moving forward, keeping track of your efforts might show you where you need to put more effort or alter your strategy. Sharing your accomplishments with a buddy or accountability partner may keep you motivated and prevent you from giving up.

Celebrate your accomplishments by keeping track of your progress. If you don't start seeing results immediately, losing weight may be a difficult process, and it can be simple to lose motivation. The minor victories along the road, Shedding a few pounds or being able to run a bit farther than before, may be seen by keeping track of your progress. Celebrating these successes may keep you inspired and constantly remind you of your progress.

Monitoring your progress is essential for losing weight. You may use it to spot trends, maintain accountability and motivation, and recognize successes. You may monitor your success in a variety of methods, such as by maintaining a food journal, keeping track of your activity, and taking progress pictures. Whatever approach you go with, remember to be patient and consistent with yourself. Although weight loss takes time, you can succeed if you are committed and persistent.

How to Hold Yourself Accountable

Greetings on starting your weight-loss journey! It may be a difficult but worthwhile experience that requires persistence and effort. Here are some guidelines for keeping oneself motivated and responsible during the procedure:

- **Realistic objectives must be made to achieve success:** These goals must also be appropriate for your lifestyle and level of fitness at the moment. An unrealistic or too-tight strategy might cause dissatisfaction and feelings of failure. Start with modest objectives and commemorate each step along the road.

- **Track your advancement:** Keeping tabs on your advancement may inspire and keep you on course. To track your daily routine, take measurements, weigh yourself often, and keep a diet and exercise log.

- **Find a support system:** When it comes to losing weight, having a support system may make all the difference. Find supportive, motivating people to be in your immediate vicinity. To help you remain accountable, consider joining a support group, hiring a personal trainer, or seeing a nutritionist.

- **Focus on forming healthy behaviors:** Instead of concentrating entirely on the number on the scale, focus on creating healthy habits. Eat a balanced diet, exercise frequently, and put self-care first.

- Being gentle with oneself is important while trying to lose weight since it is not easy. Recognize that there will be failures and obstacles; instead of beating yourself up, learn from them.

- Remember that losing weight is a process, not a final goal. You will succeed if you are persistent, determined, and driven.

Finding Support and Community

Gaining community and support is crucial to reaching weight reduction objectives. Here are some pointers to assist you in locating community and support:

- **Join a support group for people trying to lose weight:** A support group may give you a feeling of accountability and camaraderie. Sharing your experiences with others allows you to get insight from their accomplishments and failures and encouragement and support.

- **Find a workout buddy:** A buddy can keep you accountable and motivated. You may encourage one another to keep on track by sharing your fitness objectives.

- **Employ a personal trainer:** A personal trainer can offer you knowledgeable direction and support. They may inspire you, hold you responsible, and assist you in developing a specific fitness plan.

- **Connect with family and friends:** Consult with loved ones who support your efforts to lose weight. Tell them about your progress and enlist their encouragement and assistance.

- **Use social media:** Sign up for weight loss forums on websites like Facebook or Instagram. You might find motivational inspiration by connecting with others who have similar aims to your own.

Attend exercise courses at your neighborhood gym or community center. You may make new friends who have similar interests and objectives in fitness.

Finding community and support may help you remain accountable and motivated, which can help you achieve your weight reduction objectives more successfully in the long run. Feel free to contact those who can help you along the path.

Chapter 8: Overcoming Plateaus and Setbacks

Understanding Weight Loss Plateaus

When you stop losing weight while maintaining your weight reduction efforts, you have reached a weight loss plateau. Although it can be upsetting and discouraging, this is a typical aspect of the weight loss process. The following are some elements that affect weight loss plateaus:

- **Reduced metabolism:** You burn fewer calories when you lose weight because your metabolism slows down. It can make it more difficult to lose weight and cause a plateau.

- Your body could grow more adept at burning calories due to your weight reduction efforts, which might slow down weight loss.

- **Overeating:** Overeating, even for a brief time, might cause weight reduction to stall.

- **Lack of exercise:** Losing muscle mass while losing weight might cause your metabolism to slow down, making it more difficult to lose weight.

Here are some techniques that might assist you in getting through a weight loss plateau:

Check your calorie intake again to be sure you're consuming only a few or too many. Your body may enter famine mode if you consume insufficient calories, slowing your metabolism. You can ingest more calories than you burn if you consume too many.

Increase your physical activity by adding more to your daily routine. Your metabolism will increase. As a result, we are helping you burn more calories. Try a new fitness program or raise the ante on the intensity of your exercises to switch things up.

Your body may be shocked by this, breaking the plateau.

Reevaluate your objectives, It's conceivable that your aim of losing weight is no longer attainable or sustainable. Reevaluate your objectives, and make any required changes.

Practice awareness, Pay attention to your eating patterns and practice mindfulness. You may control your eating by being more aware of your body's hunger and fullness cues.

Remember that weight reduction plateaus are common, so try not to lose motivation. You may overcome the plateau and continue your weight reduction quest with a few changes to your routine.

Strategies for Breaking through Plateaus

Even though it might be difficult, going through a weight loss plateau is not impossible. Here are some tactics that might enable you to succeed:

- **Consider trying intermittent fasting:** This common eating pattern alternates between periods of fasting and eating. Through a decrease in calorie intake and an increase in fat burning, this strategy can accelerate weight loss.

- **Change up your workouts if you've been following the same routine:** Increase the intensity of your workouts and include a variety of activities.

- **Increasing your protein intake:** This will help you increase your metabolism and decrease cravings. Ensure you include foods high in protein in your diet, such as lean meats, fish, beans, and nuts.

- **Get adequate rest:** Sleep deprivation may lead to weight gain and make weight loss more difficult.

- **Control your stress:** Stress may raise your cortisol levels, which can cause you to gain weight. Add stress-reduction practices to your routine, such as yoga, meditation, or deep breathing exercises.

- Increase your water consumption to help flush out toxins, lessen bloating, and aid in weight reduction.

- **Track your progress:** Monitoring your development may keep you inspired and focused. To keep track of your progress, use a food diary, a weight loss notebook, or a monitoring app.

Remember that patience and perseverance are the keys to getting through a weight loss plateau. Maintain your efforts and maintain selecting nutritious options. You'll succeed in losing weight if you put effort into it over time.

How to Bounce Back From a Setbacks

Recovering from setbacks is a crucial component of the weight reduction process. Here are some methods that might assist you in getting back on track:

- **Determine the cause of the setback:** Step back and consider what led to the setback. Was it brought on by a particular occasion or incident, or was it a pattern of behavior? Finding the cause will enable you to create a strategy to stop it from occurring again.

- **Reframe your thinking:** See setbacks as learning opportunities rather than failures. Take advantage of setbacks to evaluate your development and make the required corrections.

- Be kind and sympathetic to yourself. Feeling disappointed after a setback is normal, so try not to be too harsh on yourself. Focus on positive self-affirmations rather than negative self-talk.

- **Reach out for assistance:** Recovering from setbacks may be easier with a support network. Contact a friend, a member of your family, or a support group for motivation and accountability.

- **Reset your objectives:** When you experience setbacks, you should review your objectives and, if required, make adjustments. Create a strategy to assist you in achieving your objectives and ensure they are both attainable and reasonable.

- **Resuming your routine: Try** to resume your wholesome routine as soon as possible. These are a few examples of planning meals, exercising, and monitoring your progress.

Setbacks are a common part of the weight reduction process. Please don't allow them to get you down or stop you from achieving your objectives. Instead, see failure as a chance to improve, learn, and keep moving.

Conclusion

Final Words of Encouragement

Congratulations on starting your weight loss journey and taking the first step toward healthy living! Making a change requires guts and tenacity. Therefore, you should be proud of yourself for acting.

You may encounter challenges and failures but remember that they are all chances to grow and learn. Celebrate your accomplishments and try not to be too harsh on yourself as you work toward a better you.

It's crucial to remember that weight reduction improves your physical look and your general health and well-being as you strive toward your objectives. Instead of relying on short-term solutions or fad diets, establish long-term lifestyle adjustments. Find a routine that works for you and stick with it because consistency is important.

Always be kind to yourself and take care of yourself as you go. Celebrate your accomplishments, no matter how minor, and don't allow failures to stop you. Make sure you have a strong network of friends, family, or a support group around you so they can help you through the highs and lows of your journey.

Last, but not least, remember that you can accomplish your objectives. Maintain your self-confidence and commitment to changing for the better. Even though your path won't be simple, it will be worthwhile. Keep moving ahead, be committed to your objectives, and have faith in your ability to succeed in anything you set out to do.

Best of luck on your weight loss journey!

www.ingramcontent.com/pod-product-compliance
Lightning Source LLC
Chambersburg PA
CBHW061514250726
48657CB00005B/1867